BANTING DIET COOKBOOK RECIPES FOR BEGINNERS

The Essential Guide to Rapid Weight Loss, Feeling Good, and a Healthy Lifestyle

Norval Ernser

Copyright

Table of Contents

Introduction

Once upon a time in the bustling city of New York, there lived a young woman named Emily. Emily was an avid reader, finding solace and inspiration within the pages of books. She possessed a unique talent - an ability to absorb knowledge effortlessly, especially when it came to cooking and nutrition.

One rainy afternoon, while browsing through the shelves of a quaint bookstore, Emily stumbled upon a book titled "BANTING DIET COOKBOOK: RECIPES FOR BEGINNERS." Intrigued by the promise of delicious recipes and healthier living, she eagerly flipped through its pages.

As Emily delved deeper into the cookbook, she found herself captivated by the principles of the Banting diet - a low-carbohydrate, high-fat eating plan designed to promote weight loss and overall wellness. With each turn of the page, she absorbed the intricacies of meal preparation, learning about nutrient-rich ingredients and innovative cooking techniques.

Armed with newfound knowledge, Emily embarked on a culinary journey unlike any other. She transformed her tiny kitchen into a bustling laboratory, experimenting with recipes that tantalized the taste buds and nourished the body.

From hearty breakfasts of avocado and bacon omelets to satisfying dinners of grilled salmon with roasted vegetables, Emily mastered the art of preparing wholesome meals that satisfied both hunger and cravings. She infused each dish with love and creativity, turning simple ingredients into culinary masterpieces.

Word of Emily's culinary prowess spread quickly throughout the neighborhood. Friends and neighbors flocked to her doorstep, eager to taste her delectable creations and learn her secrets to healthy eating. Emily graciously welcomed them into her kitchen, sharing not only her recipes but also her passion for good food and vibrant living.

As the seasons changed and the years passed, Emily's reputation as a culinary virtuoso continued to grow. She hosted cooking classes, wrote her own cookbook, and even appeared on television, spreading the gospel of the Banting diet to eager audiences far and wide.

But amidst all the accolades and recognition, Emily remained humble and grounded, always remembering the simple joy of sharing a delicious meal with loved ones. For her, cooking was more than just a skill – it was a way of life, a celebration of health, happiness, and the boundless possibilities found within the pages of a good book. And as she flipped through the well-worn pages of her beloved cookbook, Emily knew that her journey had only just begun.

Chapter 1: Understanding the Banting Diet

In recent years, the Banting Diet has emerged as a popular choice for individuals seeking to achieve rapid weight loss, improve their overall health, and adopt a sustainable lifestyle. Developed by William Banting in the 19th century and revived by Professor Tim Noakes in the modern era, the Banting Diet is grounded in the principle of low-carbohydrate, high-fat (LCHF) eating.

What is the Banting Diet?

At its core, the Banting Diet emphasizes the consumption of whole, unprocessed foods while limiting the intake of carbohydrates, particularly those with a high glycemic index. This dietary approach encourages the body to rely on fats for fuel instead of carbohydrates, a state known as ketosis.

Contrary to popular belief, the Banting Diet is not a one-size-fits-all solution. It can be tailored to suit individual preferences and nutritional needs. While some may strictly adhere to the original Banting guidelines, others may adopt a more flexible approach, incorporating elements of the diet into their existing eating habits.

Benefits of the Banting Diet

The Banting Diet offers a multitude of potential benefits, ranging from weight loss and improved metabolic health to increased energy levels and enhanced mental clarity. By reducing carbohydrate intake and increasing fat consumption, individuals may experience:

- **Weight Loss:** Lowering carbohydrate intake can lead to decreased levels of insulin, the hormone responsible for storing fat. This, in turn, promotes fat burning and facilitates weight loss.

- **Stable Blood Sugar Levels:** By minimizing fluctuations in blood sugar levels, the Banting Diet can help regulate appetite, reduce cravings, and prevent energy crashes.

- **Improved Lipid Profile:** Contrary to conventional wisdom, dietary fat is not inherently harmful. In fact, incorporating healthy fats into your diet can improve cholesterol levels and reduce the risk of cardiovascular disease.

- **Sustained Energy:** Unlike carbohydrates, which provide a quick but short-lived energy boost, fats offer a steady and prolonged source of energy, keeping you feeling satiated and energized throughout the day.

Getting Started with Banting

Embarking on a Banting journey requires a fundamental understanding of the principles underlying the diet, as well as practical strategies for implementation. Whether you're a seasoned veteran or a newcomer to the world of LCHF eating, here are some key steps to help you get started:

- **Educate Yourself:** Familiarize yourself with the basic tenets of the Banting Diet, including which foods are encouraged and which are best avoided.

- **Plan Your Meals:** Take the time to plan and prepare Banting-friendly meals and snacks in advance to ensure that you stay on track with your dietary goals.

- **Listen to Your Body:** Pay attention to how different foods make you feel and adjust your dietary choices accordingly. Everyone's nutritional needs and tolerances are unique, so it's essential to listen to your body's cues.

- **Stay Consistent:** Consistency is key to success on the Banting Diet. While occasional indulgences are perfectly normal, strive to maintain a balanced and sustainable approach to eating in the long term.

Common Misconceptions

Despite its growing popularity, the Banting Diet is not without its fair share of misconceptions and myths. It's essential to separate fact from fiction to make informed decisions about your dietary choices. Some common misconceptions about the Banting Diet include:

- It's All About Eating Bacon: While bacon is indeed a staple in many Banting recipes, the diet is not solely centered around consuming copious amounts of meat. A well-rounded Banting meal plan incorporates a variety of nutrient-dense foods, including vegetables, healthy fats, and high-quality proteins.

- It's Too Restrictive: While the Banting Diet does involve limiting certain food groups, such as grains and sugars, it still allows for a wide range of delicious and satisfying foods. With a little creativity and experimentation, you can enjoy a diverse array of Banting-friendly meals and snacks.

- It's Unsustainable in the Long Term: While some critics argue that the Banting Diet is unsustainable in the long term, many individuals have successfully adopted it as a permanent lifestyle change. By focusing on whole, unprocessed foods and listening to your body's hunger and satiety signals, you can maintain a healthy and balanced diet for years to come.

Understanding these fundamental aspects of the Banting Diet is the first step towards harnessing its transformative power and unlocking your full potential for health and wellness. As you embark on your Banting journey, remember that it's not just about achieving a specific weight loss goal—it's about embracing a sustainable lifestyle that nourishes your body, mind, and soul.

What is the Banting Diet?

The Banting Diet, also known as the LCHF (Low Carbohydrate, High Fat) diet, is a nutritional approach that emphasizes the consumption of foods low in carbohydrates and high in healthy fats. Named after William Banting, who popularized the concept in the 19th century, the Banting Diet has experienced a resurgence in recent years, championed by modern advocates like Professor Tim Noakes.

At its core, the Banting Diet challenges traditional dietary norms by prioritizing fats as the primary source of energy instead of carbohydrates. This shift in macronutrient composition induces a metabolic state known as ketosis, where the body relies on ketones—derived from fats—as its primary fuel source. By reducing carbohydrate intake and moderating protein consumption, followers of the Banting Diet aim to optimize metabolic health, promote weight loss, and improve overall well-being.

Principles of the Banting Diet:

1. Low Carbohydrate Intake: Carbohydrates, particularly those with a high glycemic index, are restricted on the Banting Diet. This includes refined sugars, grains, starchy vegetables, and most fruits. By minimizing carbohydrate intake, the diet aims to stabilize blood sugar levels and reduce insulin secretion, facilitating fat burning and weight loss.

2. Moderate Protein Consumption: While protein is an essential component of the diet, excessive intake can disrupt ketosis by stimulating the release of insulin. Therefore, the Banting Diet advocates for moderate protein consumption, focusing on high-quality sources such as lean meats, poultry, fish, and eggs.

3. Emphasis on Healthy Fats: Contrary to conventional dietary guidelines, the Banting Diet promotes the consumption of healthy fats, including monounsaturated and polyunsaturated fats found in avocados, nuts, seeds, olive oil, and fatty fish. These fats provide sustained energy, promote satiety, and support various physiological functions within the body.

4. Whole, Unprocessed Foods: The Banting Diet encourages the consumption of whole, unprocessed foods while discouraging highly refined and processed products. By prioritizing nutrient-dense foods such as leafy greens, non-starchy vegetables, nuts, seeds, and pasture-raised meats, followers of the diet aim to optimize their nutritional intake and support overall health.

Key Components of the Banting Diet:

- **Foods to Enjoy:** Non-starchy vegetables, leafy greens, avocados, nuts, seeds, coconut oil, olive oil, grass-fed meats, fatty fish, eggs, full-fat dairy products (in moderation), and select fruits low in carbohydrates (e.g., berries).

- **Foods to Avoid:** Refined sugars, grains (e.g., wheat, corn, rice), starchy vegetables (e.g., potatoes, sweet potatoes), legumes, processed foods, sugary beverages, artificial sweeteners, and most fruits high in carbohydrates (e.g., bananas, grapes, mangoes).

Benefits of the Banting Diet:

- **Weight Loss:** By promoting fat burning and reducing cravings, the Banting Diet can facilitate significant weight loss, particularly in individuals with insulin resistance or metabolic syndrome.

- **Stabilized Blood Sugar Levels:** The low-carbohydrate nature of the diet helps regulate blood sugar levels, reducing the risk of insulin spikes and crashes commonly associated with high-carb diets.

- **Improved Lipid Profile:** Contrary to traditional beliefs, consuming healthy fats can lead to favorable changes in cholesterol levels, including increased HDL ("good") cholesterol and decreased triglycerides.

- **Enhanced Mental Clarity:** Many individuals report improved cognitive function and mental clarity when following the Banting Diet, attributed to stable energy levels and reduced inflammation in the brain.

In summary, the Banting Diet represents a paradigm shift in nutritional thinking, challenging conventional wisdom about dietary fats and carbohydrates. By prioritizing whole, unprocessed foods and embracing a macronutrient balance that favors fats over carbohydrates, followers of the Banting Diet aim to achieve sustainable weight loss, improved metabolic health, and enhanced well-being.

Benefits of the Banting Diet

The Banting Diet, with its emphasis on low carbohydrate intake and high consumption of healthy fats, offers a plethora of benefits that extend beyond mere weight loss. Let's delve into some of the compelling advantages of adopting the Banting lifestyle:

1. Rapid Weight Loss:

One of the most prominent benefits of the Banting Diet is its ability to facilitate rapid and sustainable weight loss. By restricting carbohydrate intake and promoting fat burning, the body shifts from relying on glucose for energy to utilizing stored fat as fuel. This metabolic shift not only leads to a reduction in body fat but also helps curb cravings and promote feelings of satiety, making it easier to adhere to a calorie-deficient diet without feeling deprived.

2. Improved Metabolic Health:

The Banting Diet has been shown to improve various markers of metabolic health, including insulin sensitivity, blood sugar levels, and lipid profile. By reducing carbohydrate intake and stabilizing blood sugar levels, the diet can help prevent insulin spikes and crashes, reducing the risk of insulin resistance, type 2 diabetes, and metabolic syndrome. Additionally, the consumption of healthy fats can lead to favorable changes in cholesterol levels, including an increase in HDL ("good") cholesterol and a decrease in triglycerides, promoting cardiovascular health.

3. Sustained Energy Levels:

Unlike carbohydrates, which provide a quick but short-lived energy boost followed by a crash, fats offer a steady and sustained source of energy. By relying on fats for fuel, individuals following the

Banting Diet can experience consistent energy levels throughout the day, without the fluctuations commonly associated with high-carb diets. This stable energy supply not only enhances physical performance but also promotes mental clarity and focus, allowing for increased productivity and overall well-being.

4. Reduced Inflammation:

Chronic inflammation has been implicated in the development of various health conditions, including obesity, heart disease, and autoimmune disorders. The Banting Diet, with its focus on whole, unprocessed foods and anti-inflammatory fats, can help reduce inflammation levels in the body. By minimizing the consumption of inflammatory foods such as refined sugars and grains and incorporating anti-inflammatory foods such as fatty fish, nuts, and olive oil, individuals can support their body's natural defense mechanisms and promote optimal health.

5. Enhanced Satiety and Appetite Control:

One of the key challenges of traditional calorie-restricted diets is dealing with persistent hunger and cravings, which often lead to overeating and eventual weight regain. The Banting Diet addresses this issue by promoting the consumption of foods that are high in healthy fats and protein, both of which are known to increase satiety and reduce appetite. By feeling more satisfied after meals and experiencing fewer cravings, individuals following the Banting Diet can adhere to their dietary goals more effectively and achieve long-term success in weight management.

6. Improved Mental Well-being:

Emerging research suggests a link between diet and mental health, with certain dietary patterns influencing mood, cognition, and overall mental well-being. The Banting Diet, with its emphasis on nutrient-dense foods and stable energy levels, may have beneficial effects on mental health. By providing the brain with essential nutrients and promoting stable blood sugar levels, the diet can help alleviate symptoms of depression, anxiety, and cognitive decline, leading to improved mood, focus, and overall cognitive function.

The Banting Diet offers a multitude of benefits that extend far beyond weight loss. From improving metabolic health and sustaining energy levels to reducing inflammation and enhancing mental well-being, adopting a Banting lifestyle can empower individuals to take control of their health and transform their lives for the better.

Getting Started with Banting

Embarking on a Banting journey involves more than just changing what you eat; it requires a fundamental shift in mindset and approach to food. Whether you're new to the concept of low-carb, high-fat eating or looking to refine your existing dietary habits, here are some key steps to help you get started with Banting:

1. Educate Yourself:

Before diving into the Banting Diet, take the time to educate yourself about its principles, guidelines, and potential benefits. Familiarize yourself with the concept of low-carbohydrate, high-fat eating, and understand the science behind it. Resources such as books, articles, and reputable websites can provide valuable insights into the Banting lifestyle and help you make informed decisions about your dietary choices.

2. Assess Your Current Diet:

Evaluate your current dietary habits and identify areas where you can make improvements. Take note of the types and quantities of foods you typically consume, paying particular attention to your intake of carbohydrates, fats, and protein. Keep a food diary if necessary to track your eating patterns and identify potential areas for modification.

3. Clean Out Your Pantry:

Raid your pantry, refrigerator, and kitchen cabinets to remove any foods that are not compatible with the Banting Diet. This includes refined sugars, grains, processed snacks, sugary beverages, and other high-carb items. Replace these items with Banting-friendly alternatives such as healthy fats, protein-rich foods, non-starchy vegetables, and low-carb snacks.

4. Plan Your Meals:

Meal planning is key to success on the Banting Diet. Take the time to plan your meals and snacks for the week ahead, ensuring that they align with Banting principles and provide a balance of nutrients. Consider batch cooking and meal prepping to save time and effort during busy weekdays. Look for inspiration from Banting cookbooks, online recipes, and social media communities dedicated to low-carb living.

5. Stock Up on Banting Essentials:

Make a list of Banting-friendly foods and ingredients to stock up on during your next grocery trip. Focus on whole, unprocessed foods such as leafy greens, non-starchy vegetables, avocados, nuts, seeds, olive oil, coconut oil, grass-fed meats, fatty fish, eggs, and full-fat dairy products (in moderation). Be sure to read labels carefully and avoid products containing added sugars, artificial sweeteners, and other undesirable additives.

6. Stay Hydrated:

Hydration is essential for overall health and well-being, especially when following a low-carb diet like Banting. Aim to drink plenty of water throughout the day to stay hydrated and support various physiological functions within the body. Herbal teas, infused water, and sparkling water can also be enjoyable and hydrating beverage options.

7. Seek Support and Accountability:

Transitioning to a new way of eating can be challenging, so don't hesitate to seek support from friends, family, or online communities who share your Banting goals. Having a support system in place can provide encouragement, accountability, and motivation to stay on track with your dietary goals. Consider joining Banting-focused forums, social media groups, or local meetup groups to connect with like-minded individuals and share experiences and tips.

By taking these proactive steps and approaching the Banting Diet with an open mind and a commitment to self-improvement, you can set yourself up for success on your Banting journey. Remember that progress may not always be linear, and it's okay to seek guidance and make adjustments along the way. With dedication, patience, and a willingness to embrace change, you can reap the numerous benefits of the Banting lifestyle and embark on a path to better health and vitality.

Common Misconceptions

Despite its growing popularity and proven efficacy, the Banting Diet is not immune to misconceptions and myths. Let's debunk some of the most common misconceptions surrounding the Banting lifestyle:

1. It's All About Eating Bacon:

One prevalent misconception about the Banting Diet is that it revolves around consuming copious amounts of bacon and other fatty meats. While bacon is indeed a popular ingredient in many Banting recipes, the diet is not solely centered around animal products. In fact, the Banting Diet encourages a diverse and balanced approach to eating, incorporating a variety of nutrient-dense foods such as non-starchy vegetables, healthy fats, and high-quality proteins. While bacon can certainly be enjoyed in moderation, it's important to emphasize a wide range of Banting-friendly foods to ensure adequate nutrition and dietary variety.

2. It's Too Restrictive:

Another common misconception is that the Banting Diet is overly restrictive and devoid of culinary enjoyment. While the diet does involve limiting certain food groups, such as grains and sugars, it still allows for a wide range of delicious and satisfying foods. With a little creativity and experimentation, individuals following the Banting lifestyle can enjoy a diverse array of flavorful meals and snacks that cater to their taste preferences and nutritional needs. From hearty salads and savory omelets to indulgent desserts and satisfying snacks, there's no shortage of Banting-friendly options to explore and enjoy.

3. It's Unsustainable in the Long Term:

Some critics argue that the Banting Diet is unsustainable in the long term, citing concerns about nutrient deficiencies, social isolation, and potential health risks. However, many individuals have successfully adopted the Banting lifestyle as a permanent dietary choice, experiencing lasting improvements in weight management, metabolic health, and overall well-being. By focusing on whole, unprocessed foods and listening to their body's hunger and satiety signals, Banting enthusiasts can maintain a healthy and balanced diet for years to come. Additionally, with the growing availability of Banting-friendly products and resources, adhering to the diet has never been easier or more accessible.

4. It's Only for Weight Loss:

While weight loss is a common motivation for adopting the Banting Diet, it's essential to recognize that its benefits extend far beyond mere body composition changes. In addition to promoting weight loss and fat burning, the Banting lifestyle offers numerous advantages for metabolic health, energy levels, mental clarity, and overall well-being. By prioritizing nutrient-dense foods and minimizing inflammatory triggers, individuals following the Banting Diet can experience improvements in various aspects of their health, regardless of their weight loss goals.

5. It's Incompatible with Exercise:

Some people believe that the Banting Diet is incompatible with exercise, fearing that low-carb eating will impair athletic performance and recovery. However, numerous studies have shown that the Banting lifestyle can complement exercise and enhance physical performance, particularly in endurance sports and activities that rely on fat metabolism for energy. By adapting to a fat-adapted state through dietary modifications and incorporating strategic carbohydrate refeeds, athletes and fitness enthusiasts can optimize their performance and recovery while following the Banting Diet.

In summary, it's important to separate fact from fiction when it comes to the Banting Diet and approach it with an open mind and a willingness to learn. By dispelling common misconceptions and understanding the true principles and benefits of the Banting lifestyle, individuals can make informed decisions about their dietary choices and embark on a path to better health and vitality.

Chapter 2: Banting Basics: Essential Ingredients and Cooking Techniques

Understanding the foundational elements of the Banting Diet is crucial for success on your journey to better health and vitality. In this chapter, we'll explore the essential ingredients and cooking techniques that form the backbone of the Banting lifestyle.

Essential Ingredients:

1. Healthy Fats: Healthy fats are the cornerstone of the Banting Diet, providing a concentrated source of energy and essential nutrients. Incorporate a variety of healthy fats into your meals, including:

   - **Avocados:** Rich in monounsaturated fats and fiber, avocados are a versatile ingredient that adds creaminess and flavor to salads, dips, and smoothies.

- **Nuts and Seeds:** Almonds, walnuts, chia seeds, and flaxseeds are excellent sources of healthy fats, protein, and fiber. Enjoy them as snacks, or sprinkle them over salads and yogurt for added crunch and nutrition.

- **Olive Oil and Coconut Oil:** These heart-healthy oils are perfect for sautéing, roasting, and dressing salads. Opt for extra-virgin olive oil and unrefined coconut oil for maximum flavor and nutritional benefits.

2. **Quality Proteins:** Protein is essential for muscle repair, satiety, and overall health. Choose high-quality sources of protein that are rich in essential amino acids, such as:

- **Grass-fed Meats:** Grass-fed beef, lamb, and bison are leaner and contain higher levels of omega-3 fatty acids and antioxidants compared to conventionally raised meats.

- **Poultry:** Skinless chicken breasts and turkey are excellent sources of lean protein. Look for organic or free-range options whenever possible.

- **Fatty Fish:** Salmon, mackerel, trout, and sardines are rich in omega-3 fatty acids, which support heart health and brain function. Aim to include fatty fish in your diet at least twice a week.

3. **Non-Starchy Vegetables:** Non-starchy vegetables are low in carbohydrates and high in fiber, vitamins, and minerals, making them an essential component of the Banting Diet. Load up on colorful vegetables such as:

- **Leafy Greens:** Spinach, kale, arugula, and Swiss chard are nutrient powerhouses that can be enjoyed raw in salads or cooked in stir-fries and soups.

- **Cruciferous Vegetables:** Broccoli, cauliflower, Brussels sprouts, and cabbage are packed with antioxidants and phytonutrients that support detoxification and immune function.

- **Bell Peppers:** Rich in vitamin C and antioxidants, bell peppers add sweetness and crunch to dishes. Enjoy them raw with hummus or roasted in Mediterranean-inspired recipes.

Cooking Techniques:

1. Sautéing: Sautéing is a quick and versatile cooking technique that involves cooking food in a small amount of oil over medium to high heat. Use olive oil or coconut oil for sautéing vegetables, meats, and seafood, and add aromatics such as garlic, onions, and herbs for extra flavor.

2. Roasting: Roasting is a simple yet flavorful cooking method that works well for a variety of ingredients, including vegetables, meats, and seafood. Preheat your oven to the desired temperature, season your ingredients with herbs and spices, and roast them on a baking sheet until golden and tender.

3. Grilling: Grilling is a popular cooking technique that adds smoky flavor and caramelization to foods. Whether you're grilling steak, chicken, fish, or vegetables, preheat your grill to medium-high heat, oil the grates to prevent sticking, and cook your ingredients until charred and cooked through.

4. Steaming: Steaming is a gentle cooking method that preserves the natural flavors and nutrients of foods. Use a steamer basket or a steaming tray to steam vegetables, fish, and shellfish until tender and vibrant in color.

5. Stir-Frying: Stir-frying is a quick and efficient cooking technique that involves cooking small pieces of food in a hot pan or wok with a small amount of oil. Use high heat and constant stirring to cook vegetables, meats, and tofu until crisp-tender and infused with flavor.

By mastering these essential ingredients and cooking techniques, you'll be well-equipped to create delicious and satisfying meals that align with the principles of the Banting Diet. Experiment with different flavor combinations and culinary styles to keep your meals exciting and enjoyable, and don't be afraid to get creative in the kitchen!

Key Ingredients for Banting Recipes

To succeed on the Banting Diet, it's essential to stock your kitchen with a variety of nutrient-dense ingredients that align with the principles of low-carbohydrate, high-fat eating. Here are some key ingredients that form the foundation of delicious and satisfying Banting recipes:

1. Avocados: Avocados are a Banting staple, prized for their creamy texture and heart-healthy fats. They're versatile enough to be enjoyed in salads, sandwiches, dips, and smoothies, providing a rich source of monounsaturated fats, fiber, and essential nutrients like potassium and vitamin E.

2. Nuts and Seeds: Nuts and seeds are nutrient powerhouses that add crunch, flavor, and nutrition to Banting recipes. Almonds, walnuts, pecans, chia seeds, flaxseeds, and pumpkin seeds are excellent sources of healthy fats, protein, and fiber, making them ideal for snacking, baking, and topping salads and yogurt.

3. Coconut Oil: Coconut oil is a versatile cooking fat that's well-suited for high-heat cooking methods like sautéing, roasting, and frying. It contains medium-chain triglycerides (MCTs), which are readily absorbed and used by the body for energy, making it an excellent choice for Banting-friendly recipes.

4. Olive Oil: Extra-virgin olive oil is a pantry staple in many Banting households, prized for its rich flavor and heart-healthy monounsaturated fats. Use it to dress salads, drizzle over roasted vegetables, and sauté meats and seafood for added flavor and moisture.

5. Leafy Greens: Leafy greens such as spinach, kale, arugula, and Swiss chard are nutrient-dense additions to Banting recipes, providing a wealth of vitamins, minerals, and antioxidants. Incorporate them into salads, soups, stir-fries, and smoothies for a boost of fiber and flavor.

6. Grass-fed Meats: Grass-fed beef, lamb, and bison are preferred choices for Banting recipes due to their higher levels of omega-3 fatty acids, conjugated linoleic acid (CLA), and antioxidants compared to conventionally raised meats. Look for grass-fed options whenever possible to maximize flavor and nutritional benefits.

7. Fatty Fish: Fatty fish such as salmon, mackerel, trout, and sardines are excellent sources of omega-3 fatty acids, which support heart health, brain function, and inflammation regulation. Enjoy them grilled, baked, or pan-seared as part of your Banting meal plan.

8. Eggs: Eggs are a versatile and economical source of protein and essential nutrients, making them a Banting-friendly ingredient for breakfast, lunch, or dinner. Whether scrambled, poached, boiled, or baked, eggs can be enjoyed in countless savory and sweet recipes.

9. Non-Starchy Vegetables: Non-starchy vegetables such as broccoli, cauliflower, bell peppers, zucchini, and mushrooms are low in carbohydrates and high in fiber, vitamins, and minerals. They're perfect for adding volume, color, and texture to Banting recipes without spiking blood sugar levels.

10. Full-Fat Dairy Products (in Moderation): Full-fat dairy products such as cheese, yogurt, and cream can be enjoyed in moderation on the Banting Diet, providing a good source of calcium, protein, and healthy fats. Opt for organic and grass-fed options whenever possible, and choose unsweetened varieties to minimize added sugars.

By keeping these key ingredients on hand, you'll be well-prepared to create delicious and nutritious Banting recipes that support your health and wellness goals. Experiment with different flavor combinations and culinary techniques to keep your meals exciting and satisfying, and don't be afraid to get creative in the kitchen!

Cooking Techniques for Banting

Mastering cooking techniques that align with the principles of the Banting Diet is essential for creating delicious, nutrient-dense meals that support your health and wellness goals. Here are some key cooking techniques to help you elevate your Banting culinary skills:

1. **Sautéing:** Sautéing is a versatile cooking technique that involves cooking food quickly in a small amount of fat over medium to high heat. It's perfect for cooking vegetables, meats, and seafood, as it preserves their natural flavors and textures while adding depth and complexity. Use olive oil, coconut oil, or ghee for sautéing, and experiment with different aromatics like garlic, onions, and herbs to enhance the flavor of your dishes.

2. **Roasting:** Roasting is a simple yet effective cooking method that works well for a wide range of ingredients, including vegetables, meats, and

poultry. Preheat your oven to the desired temperature, season your ingredients with herbs, spices, and olive oil, and roast them on a baking sheet until golden and caramelized. Roasting intensifies the natural sweetness and depth of flavor of your ingredients, resulting in delicious and satisfying dishes that are perfect for meal prep or entertaining.

3. Grilling: Grilling is a popular cooking technique that adds smoky flavor and charred texture to foods, making it ideal for meats, fish, vegetables, and even fruits. Whether you're using a gas grill, charcoal grill, or indoor grill pan, preheat it to medium-high heat and oil the grates to prevent sticking. Grill your ingredients until they're cooked through and caramelized, flipping them halfway through cooking for even browning. Experiment with different marinades, rubs, and sauces to add flavor and variety to your grilled creations.

4. Steaming: Steaming is a gentle cooking method that preserves the natural flavors, colors, and nutrients of foods, making it ideal for vegetables, fish, and shellfish. Use a steamer basket or a steaming tray to steam your ingredients until they're tender and vibrant in color, taking care not to overcook them. Steamed vegetables can be enjoyed as a side dish or incorporated into salads, stir-fries, and grain bowls for added nutrition and texture.

5. Stir-Frying: Stir-frying is a quick and efficient cooking technique that involves cooking small pieces of food in a hot pan or wok with a small amount of oil. It's perfect for creating flavorful and colorful dishes that are packed with nutrients and texture. Use high heat and constant stirring to cook your ingredients quickly and evenly, adding aromatics like garlic, ginger, and scallions for extra flavor. Serve your stir-fries with cauliflower rice, zucchini noodles, or shirataki noodles for a low-carb alternative to traditional grains.

6. Baking: Baking is a classic cooking technique that's perfect for making a wide range of Banting-friendly dishes, including casseroles, frittatas, quiches, and desserts. Preheat your oven to the desired temperature, prepare your ingredients, and bake them in a greased baking dish or sheet pan until they're cooked through and golden brown. Experiment with different flavor combinations and ingredients to create delicious and satisfying baked goods that are perfect for any occasion.

By mastering these essential cooking techniques, you'll be well-equipped to create delicious and nutritious meals that support your health and wellness goals on the Banting Diet. Experiment with different ingredients, flavors, and culinary styles to keep your meals exciting and enjoyable, and don't be afraid to get creative in the kitchen!

Tips for Meal Prep and Planning

Meal prep and planning are essential components of success on the Banting Diet, helping you stay on track with your dietary goals and make healthier choices throughout the week. Here are some tips to streamline your meal prep and planning process:

1. *MSet Aside Time for Planning:** Dedicate a specific day or time each week to plan your meals and snacks. Take inventory of your kitchen, review your schedule for the week ahead, and decide which meals you'll prepare at home and which ones you'll eat out or order in. Having a plan in place will help you make smarter food choices and avoid last-minute temptations.

2. **Create a Meal Plan:** Use a meal planning template or app to create a weekly meal plan that includes breakfast, lunch, dinner, and snacks. Incorporate a variety of Banting-friendly ingredients and recipes, including protein-rich meats, fatty fish, non-starchy vegetables, healthy fats, and low-carb snacks. Aim for balanced meals that provide a mix of nutrients and flavors to keep you satisfied and energized throughout the day.

3. **Prep Ingredients in Advance:** Spend some time prepping ingredients in advance to save time and effort during the week. Wash, chop, and portion out vegetables, meats, and other

ingredients for recipes, and store them in airtight containers or zip-top bags in the refrigerator. Pre-cook grains, beans, and other staples to have on hand for quick and easy meals.

4. Batch Cook: Batch cooking is a time-saving strategy that involves preparing large quantities of food at once and portioning it out for multiple meals. Choose a day when you have extra time, such as the weekend, to batch cook proteins, grains, and vegetables for the week ahead. Use slow cookers, Instant Pots, and sheet pans to cook large batches of soups, stews, casseroles, and roasted vegetables with minimal effort.

5. Use Freezer-Friendly Recipes: Stock your freezer with freezer-friendly recipes that can be made in advance and reheated as needed. Soups, stews, casseroles, and baked goods are all excellent candidates for freezer storage. Portion them out into individual servings or family-sized portions, and label them with the date and contents for easy identification.

6. Invest in Meal Prep Containers: Invest in a set of high-quality meal prep containers in various sizes to store and transport your meals and snacks. Look for containers that are microwave-safe, dishwasher-safe, and BPA-free for added convenience and peace of mind. Choose containers with compartments to keep different components of your meal separate and prevent them from getting soggy or mushy.

7. Stay Flexible: While meal planning is essential for staying on track with your dietary goals, it's also important to stay flexible and adaptable to unexpected changes in your schedule or preferences. Don't be afraid to swap out ingredients, modify recipes, or improvise with what you have on hand to make meal prep and planning more manageable and enjoyable.

By incorporating these meal prep and planning tips into your routine, you'll be better equipped to stay consistent with your Banting Diet and achieve your health and wellness goals. With a little planning and preparation, you can enjoy delicious and nutritious meals that support your lifestyle and nourish your body from the inside out.

Chapter 3: Breakfasts to Kickstart Your Day

Breakfast is often hailed as the most important meal of the day, and for good reason. It sets the tone for your energy levels, mood, and overall well-being throughout the day. Here are some delicious and nutritious Banting-friendly breakfast ideas to kickstart your day on the right foot:

1. Avocado and Egg Breakfast Bowl:
   - **Ingredients:** Ripe avocado, eggs, cherry tomatoes, spinach, olive oil, salt, and pepper.
   - **Instructions:** Halve the avocado and remove the pit, creating a well in each half. Crack an egg into each avocado half and season with salt and pepper. Place them on a baking sheet and bake in a preheated oven until the eggs are set to your liking. Serve with sautéed spinach and cherry tomatoes for a nutritious and satisfying breakfast.

2. Low-Carb Veggie Omelet:

- **Ingredients:** Eggs, bell peppers, onions, mushrooms, spinach, olive oil, salt, pepper, and your choice of cheese (optional).

- **Instructions:** In a non-stick skillet, sauté diced bell peppers, onions, mushrooms, and spinach until tender. In a separate bowl, whisk eggs with salt and pepper. Pour the egg mixture into the skillet, covering the vegetables evenly. Cook until the edges are set, then sprinkle with cheese (if using) and fold the omelet in half. Cook for another minute or until the cheese is melted and the eggs are cooked through. Serve hot with a side of fresh salsa or avocado.

3. Greek Yogurt Parfait with Berries and Nuts:

- **Ingredients:** Greek yogurt, mixed berries (such as strawberries, blueberries, and raspberries), nuts (such as almonds, walnuts, or pecans), and a drizzle of honey (optional).

- **Instructions:** In a glass or bowl, layer Greek yogurt with mixed berries and nuts. Repeat the layers until you reach the top, then finish with a drizzle of honey if desired. This simple and refreshing parfait is packed with protein, fiber, and antioxidants to fuel your morning.

4. Coconut Flour Pancakes:

- **Ingredients:** Coconut flour, eggs, coconut milk, baking powder, vanilla extract, and a pinch of salt.

- **Instructions:** In a mixing bowl, whisk together coconut flour, eggs, coconut milk, baking powder, vanilla extract, and salt until smooth. Heat a non-stick skillet over medium heat and lightly grease with coconut oil. Pour the batter onto the skillet to form pancakes and cook until bubbles form on the surface, then flip and cook until golden brown on both sides. Serve with a dollop of Greek yogurt and fresh berries for a delicious and filling breakfast treat.

5. Smoked Salmon and Cream Cheese Roll-Ups:

- **Ingredients:** Smoked salmon, cream cheese, cucumber slices, avocado slices, and fresh dill (optional).

- **Instructions:** Spread a thin layer of cream cheese onto smoked salmon slices. Top with cucumber and avocado slices, then roll up tightly.

Secure with toothpicks if necessary and garnish with fresh dill. These savory roll-ups are packed with protein, healthy fats, and omega-3 fatty acids to keep you satisfied until lunchtime.

6. Green Smoothie Bowl:

- **Ingredients:** Spinach or kale, frozen banana, avocado, almond milk, protein powder (optional), and your choice of toppings (such as berries, nuts, seeds, or coconut flakes).

- **Instructions:** Blend spinach or kale, frozen banana, avocado, almond milk, and protein powder (if using) until smooth and creamy. Pour the smoothie into a bowl and top with your favorite toppings for added texture and flavor. This vibrant and nutrient-packed smoothie bowl is perfect for busy mornings when you need a quick and nourishing breakfast option.

These Banting-friendly breakfast ideas are not only delicious and satisfying but also packed with nutrients to fuel your body and mind for a productive day ahead. Experiment with different ingredients and flavors to find your favorite morning routine, and don't forget to listen to your body's hunger and satiety cues to ensure you start your day feeling energized and satisfied.

Classic Banting Breakfasts

A hearty and nutritious breakfast sets the tone for a successful day, especially on the Banting Diet. Here are some classic Banting breakfast ideas that will fuel your body and mind for the challenges ahead:

1. Bacon and Eggs:

   - **Ingredients:** Bacon strips, eggs, butter or ghee, salt, and pepper.

   - **Instructions:** Fry bacon strips until crispy in a skillet over medium heat. Remove the bacon and drain excess fat. In the same skillet, crack eggs and fry to your desired doneness in the remaining bacon fat or butter/ghee. Season with salt and pepper. Serve the eggs alongside crispy bacon for a satisfying and protein-rich breakfast.

2. Banting Breakfast Muffins:

- **Ingredients:** Eggs, spinach, bell peppers, onions, cheese (optional), salt, and pepper.

- **Instructions:** Preheat the oven to 350°F (175°C). In a mixing bowl, whisk together eggs, chopped spinach, diced bell peppers, onions, cheese (if using), salt, and pepper. Pour the mixture into greased muffin tins, filling each cup about three-quarters full. Bake for 20-25 minutes or until the muffins are set and golden brown. Enjoy these portable and protein-packed muffins for a quick and convenient breakfast on the go.

3. Smoked Salmon and Cream Cheese Bagel:

- **Ingredients:** Smoked salmon, cream cheese, cucumber slices, avocado slices, Banting-friendly bagels or cloud bread, fresh dill (optional).

- **Instructions:** Toast Banting-friendly bagels or cloud bread until golden brown. Spread a generous layer of cream cheese on each piece. Top with smoked salmon, cucumber slices, and avocado slices. Garnish with fresh dill if desired. This elegant and satisfying breakfast option is perfect for special occasions or leisurely weekend mornings.

4. Greek Yogurt with Berries and Nuts:

 - **Ingredients:** Greek yogurt, mixed berries (such as strawberries, blueberries, and raspberries), nuts (such as almonds, walnuts, or pecans), and a drizzle of honey (optional).

 - **Instructions:** In a bowl, spoon Greek yogurt and top with mixed berries and nuts. Drizzle with honey if desired. This simple and refreshing breakfast is rich in protein, fiber, and antioxidants, making it an excellent choice for busy mornings or post-workout fuel.

5. Low-Carb Breakfast Burrito:

 - **Ingredients:** Eggs, bell peppers, onions, tomatoes, avocado, cooked bacon or sausage, cheese (optional), salsa, salt, and pepper.

 - **Instructions:** In a skillet, sauté diced bell peppers, onions, and tomatoes until softened. In a separate skillet, scramble eggs until cooked through. Assemble the breakfast burrito by layering scrambled eggs, sautéed vegetables, cooked bacon or sausage, avocado slices, and cheese (if using) on a large Banting-friendly tortilla or lettuce leaf. Roll up the burrito and serve with salsa on the side. This hearty and flavorful breakfast will keep you full and satisfied until lunchtime.

These classic Banting breakfasts are not only delicious and satisfying but also packed with protein, healthy fats, and essential nutrients to fuel your body and mind for a productive day ahead. Experiment with different ingredients and flavors to create your favorite morning routine, and start your day on the right foot with a nourishing breakfast that sets you up for success.

Creative Morning Recipes

Jumpstart your mornings with these creative and flavorful Banting-friendly breakfast recipes that will tantalize your taste buds and energize your day:

1. Zucchini Fritters with Poached Eggs:
   - **Ingredients:** Zucchini, eggs, almond flour, grated Parmesan cheese, garlic powder, salt, pepper, olive oil, vinegar.
   - **Instructions:** Grate zucchini and squeeze out excess moisture. In a bowl, mix zucchini with

almond flour, Parmesan cheese, garlic powder, salt, and pepper. Form the mixture into patties and fry in olive oil until golden brown and crispy on both sides. Meanwhile, poach eggs in simmering water with a splash of vinegar. Serve the zucchini fritters topped with poached eggs for a delightful and nutritious breakfast.

2. Banting Breakfast Pizza:

- **Ingredients:** Banting-friendly pizza crust (made with almond flour or cauliflower), eggs, bacon or sausage, bell peppers, onions, cherry tomatoes, spinach, cheese (optional), salt, pepper, olive oil.

- **Instructions:** Preheat the oven according to the pizza crust recipe instructions. Prepare the pizza crust and bake until golden brown and crispy. In a skillet, cook bacon or sausage until crispy, then sauté bell peppers, onions, cherry tomatoes, and spinach until tender. Spread the cooked toppings over the baked pizza crust, crack eggs on top, and sprinkle with cheese if desired. Return to the oven and bake until the eggs are set to your liking. Slice and serve for a fun and satisfying breakfast twist.

3. Coconut Flour Waffles with Berries and Cream:

- **Ingredients:** Coconut flour, eggs, coconut milk, baking powder, vanilla extract, mixed berries (such as strawberries, blueberries, and raspberries), whipped cream (or coconut cream for dairy-free option), maple syrup or Banting-friendly sweetener.

- **Instructions:** In a bowl, whisk together coconut flour, eggs, coconut milk, baking powder, and vanilla extract until smooth. Pour the batter into a preheated waffle iron and cook until golden brown and crispy. Top the waffles with mixed berries and a dollop of whipped cream, then drizzle with maple syrup or Banting-friendly sweetener. These fluffy and indulgent waffles are perfect for weekend brunches or special occasions.

4. Egg and Bacon Breakfast Cups:

- **Ingredients:** Bacon slices, eggs, bell peppers, onions, spinach, cheese (optional), salt, pepper, cooking spray.

- **Instructions:** Preheat the oven to 375°F (190°C). Grease a muffin tin with cooking spray and line each cup with a slice of bacon. Crack an egg into each cup, then add diced bell peppers, onions, and spinach. Season with salt and pepper, and sprinkle with cheese if desired. Bake for 15-20 minutes or until the eggs are set and the bacon is crispy. Let cool slightly before removing from the muffin tin. These adorable and protein-packed breakfast cups are perfect for meal prep or on-the-go mornings.

5. Chia Seed Pudding with Almond Butter and Banana:

   - **Ingredients:** Chia seeds, almond milk, vanilla extract, almond butter, banana, sliced almonds, cinnamon, Banting-friendly sweetener (optional).

   - **Instructions:** In a jar or bowl, mix chia seeds, almond milk, and vanilla extract. Stir well and let sit for at least 30 minutes or overnight in the refrigerator until thickened. To serve, layer chia seed pudding with almond butter, sliced banana, and a sprinkle of sliced almonds and cinnamon. Drizzle with Banting-friendly sweetener if desired. This creamy and nutrient-rich pudding is a satisfying and wholesome breakfast option that's perfect for busy mornings.

Try these creative and delicious Banting breakfast recipes to add excitement and variety to your morning routine. With a balance of protein, healthy fats, and fiber-rich ingredients, these recipes will keep you fueled and satisfied until your next meal.

Energizing Smoothies and Juices

Boost your morning routine with these energizing and nutrient-packed smoothies and juices that will kickstart your day with vitality and flavor:

1. Green Goddess Smoothie:
   - **Ingredients:** Spinach, kale, cucumber, celery, green apple, lemon juice, ginger, coconut water or almond milk, ice cubes.
   - **Instructions:** In a blender, combine spinach, kale, cucumber, celery, green apple, lemon juice, ginger, coconut water or almond milk, and ice cubes. Blend until smooth and creamy. Pour into glasses and garnish with a slice of lemon or a sprig

of fresh mint. This refreshing and detoxifying green smoothie is packed with vitamins, minerals, and antioxidants to revitalize your body and mind.

2. Berry Blast Smoothie:

- **Ingredients:** Mixed berries (such as strawberries, blueberries, and raspberries), banana, spinach, Greek yogurt or coconut yogurt, almond milk, chia seeds or flaxseeds, honey or Banting-friendly sweetener (optional), ice cubes.

- **Instructions:** In a blender, combine mixed berries, banana, spinach, Greek yogurt or coconut yogurt, almond milk, chia seeds or flaxseeds, honey or Banting-friendly sweetener (if desired), and ice cubes. Blend until smooth and creamy. Pour into glasses and garnish with a few whole berries or a sprinkle of chia seeds. This vibrant and antioxidant-rich smoothie is bursting with flavor and nutrition to fuel your morning.

3. Tropical Sunshine Smoothie:

- **Ingredients:** Pineapple, mango, banana, coconut milk or coconut water, lime juice, fresh mint leaves, ice cubes.

   - **Instructions:** In a blender, combine pineapple, mango, banana, coconut milk or coconut water, lime juice, fresh mint leaves, and ice cubes. Blend until smooth and creamy. Pour into glasses and garnish with a wedge of lime or a sprig of fresh mint. This tropical-inspired smoothie is loaded with vitamin C, potassium, and electrolytes to refresh and energize your morning.

4. Citrus Zinger Juice:

   - **Ingredients:** Oranges, grapefruits, lemons, ginger, turmeric, carrots, apples, ice cubes.

   - **Instructions:** Using a juicer, juice oranges, grapefruits, lemons, ginger, turmeric, carrots, and apples. Stir the juice well to combine. Pour into glasses over ice cubes. Garnish with a slice of citrus or a sprig of fresh herbs. This zesty and invigorating juice is packed with immune-boosting vitamins, anti-inflammatory compounds, and antioxidants to kickstart your day with a burst of citrusy goodness.

5. Protein Power Smoothie:

- **Ingredients:** Protein powder (such as whey protein or plant-based protein), banana, almond butter or peanut butter, spinach or kale, almond milk or Greek yogurt, chia seeds or flaxseeds, honey or Banting-friendly sweetener (optional), ice cubes.

- **Instructions:** In a blender, combine protein powder, banana, almond butter or peanut butter, spinach or kale, almond milk or Greek yogurt, chia seeds or flaxseeds, honey or Banting-friendly sweetener (if desired), and ice cubes. Blend until smooth and creamy. Pour into glasses and garnish with a sprinkle of chia seeds or a drizzle of almond butter. This protein-packed smoothie is perfect for busy mornings or post-workout recovery, providing a balanced combination of protein, healthy fats, and carbohydrates to fuel your day.

Start your day on a refreshing and revitalizing note with these energizing smoothies and juices. Packed with vitamins, minerals, antioxidants, and protein, these breakfast options will nourish your body and invigorate your senses for a productive and vibrant day ahead.

Chapter 4: Delicious Lunches and Satisfying Dinners

Dive into a world of culinary delights with these delicious lunch and satisfying dinner recipes that will tantalize your taste buds and keep you nourished throughout the day:

Lunches:

1. Grilled Chicken Salad with Avocado Dressing:
  - **Ingredients:** Grilled chicken breast, mixed greens, cherry tomatoes, cucumber slices, avocado, red onion, olive oil, lime juice, garlic, cilantro, salt, and pepper.
  - **Instructions:** In a large bowl, combine mixed greens, cherry tomatoes, cucumber slices, and thinly sliced red onion. Top with sliced grilled chicken breast. In a blender, combine avocado, olive oil, lime juice, garlic, cilantro, salt, and pepper to make the dressing. Drizzle the dressing over the

salad and toss gently to coat. Serve immediately for a refreshing and protein-packed lunch option.

2. Zucchini Noodles with Pesto and Grilled Shrimp:

- **Ingredients:** Zucchini noodles (zoodles), grilled shrimp, homemade pesto sauce (made with basil, pine nuts, garlic, olive oil, Parmesan cheese, salt, and pepper), cherry tomatoes, grated Parmesan cheese (optional).

- **Instructions:** In a skillet, sauté zucchini noodles until tender. Toss with homemade pesto sauce until well coated. Top with grilled shrimp and halved cherry tomatoes. Sprinkle with grated Parmesan cheese if desired. This low-carb and flavorful dish is perfect for a light and satisfying lunch.

3. Turkey and Avocado Lettuce Wraps:

- **Ingredients:** Sliced turkey breast, lettuce leaves (such as romaine or butter lettuce), avocado slices, tomato slices, bacon strips, mayonnaise, mustard, salt, and pepper.

- **Instructions:** Lay lettuce leaves flat and layer with sliced turkey breast, avocado slices, tomato slices, and crispy bacon strips. Drizzle with mayonnaise and mustard, and season with salt and pepper to taste. Roll up the lettuce leaves tightly to form wraps. Serve immediately or pack them for a portable and protein-rich lunch option.

Dinners:

1. Baked Salmon with Roasted Vegetables:
   - **Ingredients:** Salmon fillets, asparagus spears, cherry tomatoes, bell peppers, red onion, olive oil, garlic, lemon zest, fresh dill, salt, and pepper.
   - **Instructions:** Preheat the oven to 400°F (200°C). Place salmon fillets on a baking sheet lined with parchment paper. Arrange asparagus spears, halved cherry tomatoes, sliced bell peppers, and thinly sliced red onion around the salmon. Drizzle with olive oil and sprinkle with minced garlic, lemon zest, fresh dill, salt, and pepper. Bake for 15-20 minutes or until the salmon is cooked through and the vegetables are tender. Serve hot with a squeeze of fresh lemon juice.

2. Banting Beef Stir-Fry with Cauliflower Rice:

- **Ingredients:** Beef strips, broccoli florets, bell peppers, carrots, snap peas, garlic, ginger, coconut aminos (or soy sauce), sesame oil, green onions, cauliflower, eggs, olive oil, salt, and pepper.

- **Instructions:** In a wok or skillet, heat olive oil over medium-high heat. Add minced garlic and ginger and cook until fragrant. Add beef strips and stir-fry until browned. Add chopped vegetables and cook until tender-crisp. Stir in coconut aminos and sesame oil, and cook for another minute. In a separate skillet, scramble eggs and stir into cauliflower rice. Serve the beef stir-fry over cauliflower rice for a flavorful and satisfying dinner option.

3. Mediterranean Stuffed Bell Peppers:

- **Ingredients:** Bell peppers, ground lamb or beef, onion, garlic, tomatoes, spinach, feta cheese, fresh parsley, dried oregano, salt, and pepper.

- **Instructions:** Preheat the oven to 375°F (190°C). Cut the tops off bell peppers and remove the seeds and membranes. In a skillet, cook ground lamb or beef with chopped onion and garlic until browned. Stir in diced tomatoes, chopped spinach, crumbled feta cheese, chopped fresh parsley, dried oregano, salt, and pepper. Spoon the mixture into the hollowed-out bell peppers. Place the stuffed peppers in a baking dish and bake for 25-30 minutes or until the peppers are tender. Serve hot with a side salad for a Mediterranean-inspired dinner.

Explore these delectable lunch and dinner recipes to add variety and flavor to your Banting meal plan. With a balance of protein, healthy fats, and colorful vegetables, these recipes are sure to satisfy your cravings and nourish your body for optimal health and wellness.

Nutrient-Packed Lunch Ideas

Elevate your midday meals with these nutrient-packed lunch ideas that are not only delicious but also nourishing and satisfying:

Nutrient-Packed Lunch Ideas:

1. Quinoa Salad with Roasted Vegetables and Chickpeas:

- **Ingredients:** Cooked quinoa, roasted vegetables (such as sweet potatoes, Brussels sprouts, and cauliflower), chickpeas, baby spinach or arugula, cherry tomatoes, red onion, feta cheese, lemon vinaigrette (made with olive oil, lemon juice, garlic, salt, and pepper).

- **Instructions:** In a large bowl, combine cooked quinoa, roasted vegetables, chickpeas, baby spinach or arugula, halved cherry tomatoes, thinly sliced red onion, and crumbled feta cheese. Drizzle with lemon vinaigrette and toss gently to coat. This vibrant and nutrient-rich salad is perfect for a light and satisfying lunch.

2. Salmon and Avocado Sushi Bowls:

- **Ingredients:** Cooked sushi rice, baked or grilled salmon fillets, avocado slices, cucumber slices, shredded carrots, nori seaweed strips, sesame seeds, soy sauce or tamari, pickled ginger, wasabi (optional).

- **Instructions:** In bowls, layer cooked sushi rice with flaked salmon, avocado slices, cucumber slices, shredded carrots, nori seaweed strips, and sesame seeds. Serve with soy sauce or tamari, pickled ginger, and wasabi on the side. These deconstructed sushi bowls are packed with omega-3 fatty acids, protein, and fiber for a satisfying and nutritious lunch option.

3. Greek-Style Chicken Pita Pockets:

- **Ingredients:** Grilled chicken breast strips, whole wheat pita bread, Greek yogurt tzatziki sauce (made with Greek yogurt, cucumber, garlic, lemon juice, dill, salt, and pepper), diced tomatoes, sliced cucumbers, red onion, Kalamata olives, feta cheese, fresh parsley.

- **Instructions:** Fill whole wheat pita pockets with grilled chicken breast strips, Greek yogurt tzatziki sauce, diced tomatoes, sliced cucumbers, thinly sliced red onion, Kalamata olives, crumbled feta cheese, and fresh parsley. These flavorful and protein-packed pita pockets are perfect for a quick and satisfying lunch on the go.

4. Vegetable and Lentil Soup:

- **Ingredients:** Brown lentils, vegetable broth, diced tomatoes, carrots, celery, onion, garlic, spinach, thyme, bay leaves, olive oil, salt, and pepper.

- **Instructions:** In a large pot, heat olive oil over medium heat. Add diced onion, carrots, and celery and cook until softened. Add minced garlic, thyme, and bay leaves and cook until fragrant. Stir in brown lentils, diced tomatoes, and vegetable broth. Bring to a boil, then reduce heat and simmer until lentils are tender. Stir in fresh spinach and season with salt and pepper to taste. This hearty and nutritious soup is packed with fiber, protein, and essential nutrients for a satisfying and comforting lunch.

5. Asian-Inspired Quinoa Bowl with Tofu:

- **Ingredients:** Cooked quinoa, baked or pan-fried tofu cubes, steamed broccoli florets, shredded cabbage, edamame beans, shredded carrots, sliced green onions, sesame seeds, soy sauce or tamari, rice vinegar, sesame oil, honey or Banting-friendly sweetener, ginger, garlic.

- **Instructions:** In bowls, layer cooked quinoa with baked or pan-fried tofu cubes, steamed broccoli florets, shredded cabbage, edamame beans, shredded carrots, and sliced green onions. In a small bowl, whisk together soy sauce or tamari, rice vinegar, sesame oil, honey or Banting-friendly sweetener, minced ginger, and minced garlic to make the dressing. Drizzle the dressing over the quinoa bowls and sprinkle with sesame seeds. These flavorful and protein-rich quinoa bowls are perfect for a nutritious and satisfying lunch.

Explore these nutrient-packed lunch ideas to add variety and flavor to your midday meals. With a balance of protein, fiber, healthy fats, and colorful vegetables, these recipes are sure to keep you fueled and satisfied throughout the day.

Flavorful Dinner Recipes

Indulge in a culinary adventure with these flavorful dinner recipes that are sure to impress your taste buds and satisfy your hunger:

Flavorful Dinner Recipes:

1. Creamy Garlic Parmesan Chicken:

- **Ingredients:** Chicken breasts, garlic cloves, fresh thyme, chicken broth, heavy cream, Parmesan cheese, butter, olive oil, salt, and pepper.

- **Instructions:** Season chicken breasts with salt and pepper. In a skillet, heat olive oil over medium-high heat and brown chicken on both sides until golden. Remove chicken from the skillet and set aside. In the same skillet, melt butter and sauté minced garlic until fragrant. Add fresh thyme, chicken broth, and heavy cream. Bring to a simmer, then return chicken to the skillet. Cook until chicken is cooked through and sauce has thickened. Stir in grated Parmesan cheese until melted and creamy. Serve hot with your favorite side dishes.

2. Mushroom and Spinach Stuffed Chicken Breast:

- **Ingredients:** Chicken breasts, baby spinach, mushrooms, garlic, cream cheese, Parmesan cheese, olive oil, salt, and pepper.

- **Instructions:** Preheat the oven to 375°F (190°C). In a skillet, heat olive oil over medium heat and sauté minced garlic until fragrant. Add sliced mushrooms and cook until tender. Stir in baby spinach and cook until wilted. Remove from heat and let cool slightly. In a bowl, mix cooked mushrooms and spinach with cream cheese and grated Parmesan cheese. Cut a pocket in each chicken breast and stuff with the mushroom-spinach mixture. Season the outside of the chicken breasts with salt and pepper. Place stuffed chicken breasts on a baking sheet lined with parchment paper and bake for 25-30 minutes or until chicken is cooked through. Serve hot with steamed vegetables or a side salad.

3. Spaghetti Squash with Turkey Meatballs and Marinara Sauce:

- **Ingredients:** Spaghetti squash, ground turkey, onion, garlic, Italian seasoning, breadcrumbs (or almond flour for low-carb option), egg, marinara sauce, olive oil, salt, and pepper.

- **Instructions:** Preheat the oven to 400°F (200°C). Cut spaghetti squash in half lengthwise and scoop out the seeds. Place squash halves cut side down on a baking sheet lined with parchment paper. Bake for 40-45 minutes or until tender. Meanwhile, in a bowl, mix together ground turkey, finely chopped onion, minced garlic, Italian seasoning, breadcrumbs or almond flour, egg, salt, and pepper. Form the mixture into meatballs and place them on a separate baking sheet. Bake meatballs for 20-25 minutes or until cooked through. Heat marinara sauce in a skillet and add cooked meatballs to the sauce. Using a fork, scrape the flesh of the cooked spaghetti squash into strands. Serve spaghetti squash topped with turkey meatballs and marinara sauce. Garnish with grated Parmesan cheese and fresh basil if desired.

4. Banting Beef Curry with Cauliflower Rice:

- **Ingredients:** Beef stew meat, onion, garlic, ginger, curry powder, turmeric, cumin, coriander, cinnamon, tomatoes, coconut milk, cauliflower, olive oil, salt, and pepper.

- **Instructions:** In a large pot, heat olive oil over medium heat and sauté diced onion until translucent. Add minced garlic and grated ginger and cook until fragrant. Stir in curry powder, turmeric, cumin, coriander, and cinnamon. Add beef stew meat and cook until browned on all sides. Add diced tomatoes and coconut milk, and bring to a simmer. Cover and cook for 1.5-2 hours or until beef is tender. Meanwhile, pulse cauliflower florets in a food processor until they resemble rice grains. Heat olive oil in a skillet and sauté cauliflower rice until tender. Season with salt and pepper. Serve beef curry over cauliflower rice for a flavorful and satisfying dinner.

5. Stuffed Bell Peppers with Quinoa and Black Beans:

- **Ingredients:** Bell peppers, cooked quinoa, black beans, corn kernels, diced tomatoes, onion, garlic, chili powder, cumin, paprika, shredded cheese (such as cheddar or Monterey Jack), fresh cilantro, olive oil, salt, and pepper.

- **Instructions:** Preheat the oven to 375°F (190°C). Cut the tops off bell peppers and remove the seeds and membranes. In a skillet, heat olive oil over medium heat and sauté diced onion until translucent. Add minced garlic and cook until fragrant. Stir in cooked quinoa, black beans, corn kernels, diced tomatoes, chili powder, cumin, paprika, salt, and pepper. Cook for 5-7 minutes or until heated through. Remove from heat and stir in shredded cheese and chopped fresh cilantro. Stuff the bell peppers with the quinoa mixture and place them in a baking dish. Cover with aluminum foil and bake for 30-35 minutes or until peppers are tender. Serve hot with additional cheese and cilantro for garnish.

Explore these flavorful dinner recipes to add excitement and variety to your evening meals. With a balance of protein, vegetables, and spices, these recipes are sure to delight your taste buds and satisfy your cravings for a delicious and satisfying dinner.

Banting-Friendly Side Dishes

Complement your main courses with these Banting-friendly side dishes that are both delicious and satisfying:

Banting-Friendly Side Dishes:

1. Roasted Garlic Cauliflower Mash:

 - **Ingredients:** Cauliflower, garlic cloves, olive oil, salt, and pepper.

 - **Instructions:** Preheat the oven to 400°F (200°C). Cut cauliflower into florets and toss with whole garlic cloves, olive oil, salt, and pepper. Spread onto a baking sheet and roast for 25-30 minutes or until cauliflower is tender and golden brown. Transfer roasted cauliflower and garlic to a food processor and blend until smooth. Adjust seasoning if necessary. Serve hot as a flavorful and low-carb alternative to mashed potatoes.

2. Sauteed Spinach with Garlic and Lemon:

 - **Ingredients:** Fresh spinach, garlic cloves, olive oil, lemon juice, salt, and pepper.

 - **Instructions:** Heat olive oil in a skillet over medium heat. Add minced garlic and cook until fragrant. Add fresh spinach leaves and cook until wilted. Remove from heat and drizzle with lemon juice. Season with salt and pepper to taste. Serve hot as a vibrant and nutritious side dish.

3. Grilled Asparagus with Parmesan Cheese:

- **Ingredients:** Asparagus spears, olive oil, grated Parmesan cheese, lemon zest, salt, and pepper.

- **Instructions:** Preheat the grill to medium-high heat. Toss asparagus spears with olive oil, salt, and pepper. Grill for 4-5 minutes per side or until tender and charred. Remove from grill and sprinkle with grated Parmesan cheese and lemon zest. Serve hot as a flavorful and elegant side dish.

4. Cucumber Tomato Salad with Balsamic Dressing:

- **Ingredients:** Cucumbers, tomatoes, red onion, fresh basil leaves, olive oil, balsamic vinegar, salt, and pepper.

- **Instructions:** Slice cucumbers, tomatoes, and red onion thinly. Tear fresh basil leaves into small pieces. In a bowl, toss sliced vegetables and basil with olive oil, balsamic vinegar, salt, and pepper. Let marinate for at least 10 minutes before serving. Serve chilled as a refreshing and colorful side dish.

5. Sauteed Brussels Sprouts with Bacon and Balsamic Glaze:

- **Ingredients:** Brussels sprouts, bacon strips, olive oil, balsamic glaze, salt, and pepper.

- **Instructions:** Cook bacon strips in a skillet until crispy. Remove bacon from skillet and chop into pieces. Trim and halve Brussels sprouts. In the same skillet with bacon drippings, add halved Brussels sprouts and cook until tender and caramelized. Season with salt and pepper. Add chopped bacon back to the skillet and toss to combine. Drizzle with balsamic glaze before serving. Serve hot as a savory and satisfying side dish.

6. Zucchini Noodles with Pesto Sauce:

- **Ingredients:** Zucchini, olive oil, homemade pesto sauce (made with basil, pine nuts, garlic, olive oil, Parmesan cheese, salt, and pepper).

- **Instructions:** Using a spiralizer, create zucchini noodles (zoodles). Heat olive oil in a skillet over medium heat and sauté zucchini noodles until tender. Toss with homemade pesto sauce until well coated. Serve hot as a flavorful and low-carb side dish.

These Banting-friendly side dishes are perfect for complementing your main courses and adding variety to your meals. Packed with flavor and nutrition, these recipes will elevate your dining experience and keep you satisfied and nourished.

Chapter 5: Irresistible Snacks and Desserts

Indulge your cravings with these irresistible snacks and desserts that are sure to satisfy your sweet tooth and keep you energized throughout the day:

Irresistible Snacks:

1. Cheese and Charcuterie Board:
   - **Ingredients:** Assorted cheeses (such as brie, cheddar, and gouda), cured meats (such as prosciutto, salami, and chorizo), olives, nuts (such as almonds, walnuts, and pistachios), sliced vegetables (such as cucumber, bell peppers, and cherry tomatoes), crackers (choose Banting-friendly options).
   - **Instructions:** Arrange assorted cheeses, cured meats, olives, nuts, sliced vegetables, and crackers on a serving board or platter. Serve as a delicious and satisfying snack for entertaining or a cozy night in.

2. Avocado and Tomato Salsa with Crispy Tortilla Chips:

- **Ingredients:** Ripe avocados, tomatoes, red onion, cilantro, lime juice, salt, pepper, corn tortillas.

- **Instructions:** In a bowl, mash ripe avocados with diced tomatoes, finely chopped red onion, chopped cilantro, lime juice, salt, and pepper to make the salsa. Cut corn tortillas into wedges, brush with olive oil, and sprinkle with salt. Bake in the oven at 350°F (175°C) until crispy. Serve the avocado and tomato salsa with crispy tortilla chips for a flavorful and satisfying snack.

3. Bacon-Wrapped Jalapeño Poppers:

- **Ingredients:** Jalapeño peppers, cream cheese, shredded cheddar cheese, bacon slices.

- **Instructions:** Preheat the oven to 400°F (200°C). Cut jalapeño peppers in half lengthwise and remove the seeds and membranes. In a bowl, mix cream cheese with shredded cheddar cheese. Fill each jalapeño half with the cheese mixture. Wrap each jalapeño half with a bacon slice and secure with toothpicks. Place on a baking sheet lined with parchment paper and bake for 20-25 minutes or until bacon is crispy and jalapeños are tender. Serve hot as a spicy and indulgent snack.

Irresistible Desserts:

1. Chocolate Avocado Mousse:

- **Ingredients:** Ripe avocados, cocoa powder, honey or Banting-friendly sweetener, vanilla extract, almond milk (optional), dark chocolate shavings (optional).

- **Instructions:** In a blender or food processor, blend ripe avocados with cocoa powder, honey or Banting-friendly sweetener, vanilla extract, and almond milk (if needed) until smooth and creamy. Adjust sweetness to taste. Spoon the chocolate avocado mousse into serving glasses and garnish with dark chocolate shavings if desired. Chill in the refrigerator for at least 30 minutes before serving. This rich and creamy dessert is a guilt-free indulgence.

2. Berry Chia Seed Pudding Parfait:

- **Ingredients:** Mixed berries (such as strawberries, blueberries, and raspberries), chia seeds, almond milk, honey or Banting-friendly sweetener, Greek yogurt or coconut yogurt, granola (choose Banting-friendly options).

- **Instructions:** In a jar or bowl, mix chia seeds with almond milk and honey or Banting-friendly sweetener. Stir well and let sit in the refrigerator for at least 2 hours or overnight until thickened. To assemble the parfait, layer chia seed pudding with Greek yogurt or coconut yogurt, mixed berries, and granola in serving glasses or jars. Repeat layers until glasses are filled. Serve chilled as a refreshing and nutritious dessert.

3. Almond Flour Lemon Bars:

- **Ingredients:** Almond flour, butter, powdered erythritol or Banting-friendly sweetener, eggs, lemon zest, lemon juice, baking powder, salt.

- **Instructions:** Preheat the oven to 350°F (175°C). In a mixing bowl, combine almond flour, melted butter, powdered erythritol or Banting-friendly sweetener, and a pinch of salt to make the crust. Press the crust mixture into the bottom of a greased baking dish and bake for 10-12 minutes or until lightly golden. In another bowl, whisk together eggs, lemon zest, lemon juice, baking powder, and a pinch of salt to make the lemon filling. Pour the lemon filling over the baked crust and return to the oven. Bake for another 20-25 minutes or until the filling is set. Let cool before slicing into bars. These tangy and sweet lemon bars are a delightful treat for any occasion.

4. Coconut Flour Chocolate Chip Cookies:

- **Ingredients:** Coconut flour, coconut oil, eggs, honey or Banting-friendly sweetener, vanilla extract, dark chocolate chips.

- **Instructions:** Preheat the oven to 350°F (175°C). In a mixing bowl, combine coconut flour, melted coconut oil, eggs, honey or Banting-friendly sweetener, and vanilla extract until a dough forms. Fold in dark chocolate chips. Roll the dough into balls and flatten slightly onto a baking sheet lined with parchment paper. Bake for 12-15 minutes or until edges are golden brown. Let cool before serving. These soft and chewy coconut flour chocolate chip cookies are a delicious and wholesome treat.

Indulge in these irresistible snacks and desserts to satisfy your cravings and treat yourself to a moment of bliss. With a balance of flavors and textures, these recipes are sure to delight your taste buds and leave you wanting more.

Guilt-Free Snack Options

Satisfy your cravings without the guilt with these wholesome and delicious snack options that are perfect for any time of the day:

Guilt-Free Snack Options:

1. Crispy Kale Chips:
 - **Ingredients:** Fresh kale leaves, olive oil, salt, and pepper.
 - **Instructions:** Preheat the oven to 275°F (135°C). Wash and thoroughly dry kale leaves, then tear them into bite-sized pieces, discarding the tough stems. Toss the kale pieces with olive oil,

salt, and pepper until evenly coated. Spread the kale in a single layer on a baking sheet lined with parchment paper. Bake for 20-25 minutes, or until the kale is crispy but not burnt. Let cool before serving. These crunchy kale chips are packed with vitamins and minerals, making them a guilt-free alternative to potato chips.

2. Cucumber Slices with Hummus:

- **Ingredients:** Cucumber, hummus (choose Banting-friendly options).

- **Instructions:** Wash and slice a cucumber into rounds. Serve the cucumber slices with a side of hummus for dipping. Cucumbers are low in calories and high in water content, while hummus provides protein and healthy fats, making this snack option both refreshing and satisfying.

3. Roasted Chickpeas:

- **Ingredients:** Canned chickpeas (garbanzo beans), olive oil, salt, and spices of your choice (such as paprika, cumin, or garlic powder).

- **Instructions:** Preheat the oven to 400°F (200°C). Rinse and drain canned chickpeas, then pat them dry with a clean kitchen towel. Toss the chickpeas with olive oil, salt, and your choice of spices until evenly coated. Spread the chickpeas in a single layer on a baking sheet lined with parchment paper. Roast for 25-30 minutes, shaking the pan halfway through, until the chickpeas are crispy and golden brown. Let cool before serving. These roasted chickpeas are crunchy and flavorful, providing a satisfying crunch without the guilt.

4. Greek Yogurt with Berries and Almonds:

   - **Ingredients:** Greek yogurt, mixed berries (such as strawberries, blueberries, and raspberries), almonds.

   - **Instructions:** Spoon Greek yogurt into a bowl and top with mixed berries and a handful of almonds. Greek yogurt is high in protein and probiotics, while berries are packed with antioxidants and fiber. Almonds add a satisfying crunch and healthy fats, making this snack option both nutritious and delicious.

5. Stuffed Medjool Dates:

- **Ingredients:** Medjool dates, almond butter or peanut butter, unsweetened shredded coconut, dark chocolate chips.

- **Instructions:** Pit Medjool dates and slice them lengthwise. Fill each date with a dollop of almond butter or peanut butter, then sprinkle with unsweetened shredded coconut and dark chocolate chips. Medjool dates are naturally sweet and rich in fiber, while almond butter or peanut butter provides protein and healthy fats. This decadent snack satisfies your sweet cravings while providing a nutritious boost.

6. Apple Slices with Almond Butter:

- **Ingredients:** Apple, almond butter.

- **Instructions:** Wash and slice an apple into wedges. Serve the apple slices with a side of almond butter for dipping. Apples are high in fiber and vitamins, while almond butter adds protein and healthy fats, making this snack option both satisfying and wholesome.

Enjoy these guilt-free snack options whenever you need a quick and nutritious pick-me-up. With a balance of flavors and nutrients, these snacks will keep you energized and satisfied throughout the day.

Indulgent Banting Desserts

Treat yourself to decadent indulgence with these Banting-friendly dessert recipes that are sure to satisfy your sweet cravings without compromising on flavor:

Indulgent Banting Desserts:

1. Dark Chocolate Avocado Truffles:

- **Ingredients:** Ripe avocados, dark chocolate (at least 70% cocoa), cocoa powder, Banting-friendly sweetener (such as erythritol or stevia), vanilla extract, salt.

- **Instructions:**

1. Melt dark chocolate in a double boiler or microwave, stirring until smooth.

2. In a blender or food processor, blend ripe avocados until creamy.

3. Add melted chocolate, cocoa powder, Banting-friendly sweetener, vanilla extract, and a pinch of salt to the blender. Blend until well combined and smooth.

4. Chill the mixture in the refrigerator for 1-2 hours, or until firm enough to handle.

5. Roll the chilled mixture into small balls and coat with cocoa powder.

6. Serve chilled and enjoy these rich and creamy chocolate truffles as a luxurious Banting-friendly dessert.

2. Low-Carb Cheesecake with Almond Crust:

- **Ingredients:** Almond flour, butter, cream cheese, Banting-friendly sweetener (such as erythritol or stevia), eggs, vanilla extract, lemon zest, sour cream.

- **Instructions:**

1. Preheat the oven to 325°F (160°C). Grease a springform pan and line the bottom with parchment paper.

2. In a mixing bowl, combine almond flour, melted butter, and a pinch of salt to make the crust.

Press the crust mixture into the bottom of the prepared pan.

3. In another mixing bowl, beat cream cheese with Banting-friendly sweetener until smooth. Add eggs one at a time, beating well after each addition. Stir in vanilla extract, lemon zest, and sour cream until well combined.

4. Pour the cream cheese mixture over the crust in the pan. Smooth the top with a spatula.

5. Bake for 40-45 minutes, or until the edges are set and the center is slightly jiggly.

6. Let the cheesecake cool in the pan for 1 hour, then refrigerate for at least 4 hours or overnight before serving. Serve chilled with your favorite Banting-friendly toppings, such as fresh berries or whipped cream.

3. Coconut Flour Chocolate Cake:

- **Ingredients:** Coconut flour, cocoa powder, Banting-friendly sweetener (such as erythritol or stevia), baking powder, salt, eggs, coconut milk, coconut oil, vanilla extract.

- **Instructions:**

1. Preheat the oven to 350°F (175°C). Grease a cake pan and line the bottom with parchment paper.

2. In a mixing bowl, whisk together coconut flour, cocoa powder, Banting-friendly sweetener, baking powder, and salt.

3. In another mixing bowl, beat eggs with coconut milk, melted coconut oil, and vanilla extract until well combined.

4. Gradually add the dry ingredients to the wet ingredients, mixing until smooth and well combined.

5. Pour the batter into the prepared cake pan and spread it evenly.

6. Bake for 25-30 minutes, or until a toothpick inserted into the center comes out clean.

7. Let the cake cool in the pan for 10 minutes, then transfer to a wire rack to cool completely.

8. Serve slices of this moist and decadent coconut flour chocolate cake as a delightful Banting-friendly dessert.

4. Almond Butter Blondies:

- **Ingredients:** Almond butter, Banting-friendly sweetener (such as erythritol or stevia), eggs, almond flour, baking powder, vanilla extract, salt, dark chocolate chips (optional).

- Instructions:

1. Preheat the oven to 350°F (175°C). Grease a baking dish and line it with parchment paper.

2. In a mixing bowl, beat almond butter with Banting-friendly sweetener until smooth.

3. Add eggs one at a time, beating well after each addition. Stir in almond flour, baking powder, vanilla extract, and a pinch of salt until well combined.

4. Fold in dark chocolate chips if desired.

5. Pour the batter into the prepared baking dish and spread it evenly.

6. Bake for 20-25 minutes, or until the top is golden brown and a toothpick inserted into the center comes out clean.

7. Let the blondies cool in the pan for 10 minutes, then transfer to a wire rack to cool completely.

8. Cut into squares and enjoy these chewy and nutty almond butter blondies as a guilt-free Banting-friendly dessert.

Indulge in these indulgent Banting desserts for a delightful and satisfying treat without the guilt. With a balance of wholesome ingredients and decadent flavors, these desserts are sure to become your new favorites.

Sweet Treats for Any Occasion

Satisfy your sweet tooth with these delectable treats suitable for any occasion. From quick snacks to elegant desserts, these recipes are sure to please:

Sweet Treats for Any Occasion:

1. Chocolate Peanut Butter Energy Balls:
   - **Ingredients:** Rolled oats, peanut butter, honey or maple syrup, cocoa powder, chocolate chips (optional), vanilla extract.
   - **Instructions:**
     1. In a mixing bowl, combine rolled oats, peanut butter, honey or maple syrup, cocoa powder, chocolate chips (if using), and vanilla extract.

2. Mix until well combined and the mixture holds together when pressed.

3. Roll the mixture into bite-sized balls and place them on a baking sheet lined with parchment paper.

4. Chill in the refrigerator for at least 30 minutes before serving.

5. Enjoy these chocolate peanut butter energy balls as a nutritious and delicious snack any time of the day.

2. Banana Bread Muffins:

- **Ingredients:** Ripe bananas, almond flour, eggs, Banting-friendly sweetener (such as erythritol or stevia), baking powder, cinnamon, vanilla extract, chopped nuts (optional).

- **Instructions:**

1. Preheat the oven to 350°F (175°C). Grease a muffin tin or line it with paper liners.

2. In a mixing bowl, mash ripe bananas until smooth. Add almond flour, eggs, Banting-friendly sweetener, baking powder, cinnamon, vanilla extract, and chopped nuts (if using).

3. Mix until well combined.

4. Divide the batter evenly among the muffin cups.

5. Bake for 20-25 minutes, or until a toothpick inserted into the center comes out clean.

6. Let the muffins cool in the tin for 5 minutes before transferring them to a wire rack to cool completely.

7. Serve these banana bread muffins warm or at room temperature for a comforting and satisfying treat.

3. Raspberry Coconut Chia Pudding:

- **Ingredients:** Chia seeds, coconut milk, raspberries, Banting-friendly sweetener (such as erythritol or stevia), vanilla extract, shredded coconut.

- **Instructions:**

1. In a mixing bowl, combine chia seeds, coconut milk, Banting-friendly sweetener, and vanilla extract.

2. Mix well and let sit in the refrigerator for at least 2 hours or overnight, stirring occasionally, until thickened.

3. In a separate bowl, mash raspberries with a fork until smooth.

4. To assemble the chia pudding, layer chia seed mixture and mashed raspberries in serving glasses.

5. Top with shredded coconut.

6. Serve chilled as a refreshing and nutritious dessert or snack.

4. Almond Flour Blueberry Crisp:

- **Ingredients:** Blueberries, almond flour, Banting-friendly sweetener (such as erythritol or stevia), lemon juice, cinnamon, salt, butter or coconut oil, chopped nuts (such as almonds or pecans).

- **Instructions:**

1. Preheat the oven to 350°F (175°C). Grease a baking dish.

2. In a mixing bowl, toss blueberries with lemon juice, Banting-friendly sweetener, cinnamon, and a pinch of salt.

3. Transfer the blueberry mixture to the prepared baking dish.

4. In another mixing bowl, combine almond flour, Banting-friendly sweetener, and chopped nuts. Mix well.

5. Cut in butter or coconut oil until the mixture resembles coarse crumbs.

6. Sprinkle the almond flour mixture over the blueberries in the baking dish.

7. Bake for 30-35 minutes, or until the topping is golden brown and the blueberries are bubbling.

8. Let cool slightly before serving.

9. Serve this almond flour blueberry crisp warm with a dollop of Greek yogurt or whipped cream for a delightful dessert.

5. Coconut Flour Lemon Bars:

- **Ingredients:** Coconut flour, butter or coconut oil, Banting-friendly sweetener (such as erythritol or stevia), eggs, lemon zest, lemon juice, baking powder, salt.

- **Instructions:**

1. Preheat the oven to 350°F (175°C). Grease a baking dish and line it with parchment paper.

2. In a mixing bowl, combine coconut flour, melted butter or coconut oil, Banting-friendly sweetener, and a pinch of salt to make the crust.

3. Press the crust mixture into the bottom of the prepared baking dish.

4. In another mixing bowl, whisk together eggs, lemon zest, lemon juice, baking powder, and a pinch of salt to make the lemon filling.

5. Pour the lemon filling over the crust in the baking dish.

6. Bake for 20-25 minutes, or until the filling is set and the edges are lightly golden.

7. Let cool in the pan for 10 minutes, then transfer to a wire rack to cool completely.

8. Cut into squares and serve these coconut flour lemon bars as a zesty and refreshing dessert.

Enjoy these sweet treats for any occasion, whether you're hosting a gathering or simply treating yourself to a delicious snack. With a balance of flavors and textures, these recipes are sure to delight your taste buds and satisfy your cravings.

Appendix: Additional Resources and Tools

Enhance your Banting journey with these additional resources and tools to support your success and help you achieve your health and wellness goals:

1. Banting Recipe Books: Explore a variety of Banting recipe books available in stores or online, offering a wide range of delicious and nutritious meal ideas to keep your diet interesting and enjoyable.

2. Online Banting Communities: Join online forums, social media groups, or communities dedicated to the Banting lifestyle. Connect with like-minded individuals, share experiences, ask questions, and find inspiration from others on similar journeys.

3. Banting Apps: Utilize Banting-focused mobile apps designed to track your food intake, monitor your progress, discover new recipes, and access helpful resources on the go. These apps can provide valuable support and guidance throughout your Banting journey.

4. Nutritional Guides: Refer to reputable nutritional guides and resources that offer information on Banting-approved foods, portion sizes, macronutrient ratios, and tips for maintaining a balanced and healthy diet while following the Banting principles.

5. Cooking Classes and Workshops: Attend cooking classes or workshops specifically tailored to Banting cooking techniques and recipes. Learn new culinary skills, discover creative meal ideas, and gain confidence in preparing delicious and nutritious Banting-friendly dishes at home.

6. Meal Planning Templates: Use meal planning templates and tools to organize your weekly meals, create shopping lists, and ensure you have all the ingredients you need to prepare Banting-approved meals ahead of time. Meal planning can help save time, reduce stress, and support consistency in your dietary habits.

7. Fitness Programs: Incorporate regular physical activity into your Banting lifestyle by exploring fitness programs, workout routines, or exercise classes that align with your preferences and fitness goals. Regular exercise can enhance the benefits of the Banting diet and contribute to overall health and well-being.

8. Educational Resources: Stay informed and educated about the science behind the Banting diet, its principles, and potential health benefits by accessing reliable educational resources such as books, articles, podcasts, and online courses written or endorsed by experts in the field.

By utilizing these additional resources and tools, you can optimize your Banting experience, stay motivated and informed, and cultivate a sustainable and fulfilling approach to healthy living. Remember to listen to your body, make adjustments as needed, and celebrate your progress along the way.

Banting Diet Resources

Explore these valuable resources and tools specifically tailored to support your Banting diet journey and help you achieve your health and wellness goals:

1. Banting Websites and Blogs: Discover reputable websites and blogs dedicated to the Banting lifestyle, offering a wealth of information, recipes, success stories, and tips to help you navigate the Banting diet with ease.

2. Banting Food Lists: Access comprehensive food lists outlining Banting-approved foods, including proteins, vegetables, fats, and fruits, to help you make informed choices and create balanced meals that align with the Banting principles.

3. Banting Recipe Websites: Explore online platforms featuring a wide range of Banting-friendly recipes, from breakfasts and main dishes to snacks and desserts, providing you with endless inspiration and creativity in the kitchen.

4. Banting Cookbooks: Invest in Banting cookbooks authored by reputable experts in the field, offering a collection of delicious and nutritious recipes that adhere to Banting guidelines, making meal planning and preparation simple and enjoyable.

5. Banting Apps: Download Banting-specific mobile apps that offer meal planning tools, recipe databases, shopping lists, and tracking features to help you stay organized, motivated, and on track with your Banting diet goals.

6. Banting Support Groups: Join local or online support groups and communities focused on the Banting diet, where you can connect with others, share experiences, seek advice, and find encouragement and motivation on your Banting journey.

7. Banting Seminars and Workshops: Attend seminars, workshops, or webinars conducted by Banting experts, where you can deepen your understanding of the Banting diet, learn practical tips, and engage in discussions with like-minded individuals.

8. Banting Health Practitioners: Consult with qualified health practitioners, such as dietitians, nutritionists, or healthcare professionals, who specialize in the Banting diet and can provide personalized guidance and support based on your individual needs and goals.

9. Banting Social Media Accounts: Follow reputable Banting advocates, chefs, and influencers on social media platforms for daily inspiration, recipe ideas, tips, and updates on the latest trends and developments in the Banting community.

10. Banting Online Courses: Enroll in online courses or programs that offer in-depth education and guidance on the Banting diet, including its principles, benefits, meal planning strategies, and practical tips for long-term success.

By utilizing these Banting diet resources and tools, you can enhance your understanding of the Banting lifestyle, access valuable support and guidance, and empower yourself to make informed choices that promote health, well-being, and vitality.

Helpful Kitchen Gadgets

Equip your kitchen with these helpful gadgets and tools designed to streamline meal preparation, enhance culinary creativity, and support your Banting diet journey:

1. Spiralizer: Transform vegetables like zucchini, carrots, and sweet potatoes into noodles or "zoodles" with a spiralizer. Create low-carb alternatives to pasta dishes and add variety to your meals with ease.

2. Food Processor: Speed up meal prep and effortlessly blend, chop, and puree ingredients with a food processor. Use it to make homemade sauces, dips, nut butters, and desserts without the hassle of manual chopping or blending.

3. Blender: Whip up nutritious smoothies, creamy soups, and homemade sauces with a high-speed blender. Blend together fresh fruits, leafy greens, and protein sources for quick and convenient meals or snacks.

4. Air Fryer: Enjoy crispy and delicious foods with less oil by using an air fryer. Cook Banting-friendly snacks like crispy kale chips, chicken wings, or roasted vegetables for a healthier alternative to traditional frying methods.

5. Immersion Blender: Easily blend soups, sauces, and smoothies directly in the pot or container with an immersion blender. Its compact size and versatility make it a convenient tool for quick and mess-free blending.

6. Vegetable Steamer: Preserve the nutrients and natural flavors of vegetables by steaming them with a vegetable steamer. Steam a variety of vegetables to accompany your meals or incorporate them into Banting-friendly recipes.

7. Cast Iron Skillet: Cook meats, vegetables, and eggs to perfection with a durable and versatile cast iron skillet. Its superior heat retention and non-stick surface make it ideal for searing, sautéing, and frying Banting-approved ingredients.

8. Food Scale: Accurately measure ingredients and portion sizes with a digital food scale. Maintain portion control and track your intake of proteins, fats, and carbohydrates to stay on track with your Banting diet goals.

9. Mandoline Slicer: Achieve uniform slices of fruits and vegetables with a mandoline slicer. Create thin slices for salads, gratins, or vegetable chips, allowing for even cooking and presentation in your dishes.

10. Instant Pot: Prepare flavorful and nutritious meals in a fraction of the time with an Instant Pot. This multi-functional pressure cooker can sauté, steam, slow cook, and more, offering endless possibilities for Banting-friendly recipes.

Investing in these helpful kitchen gadgets can simplify meal preparation, inspire culinary creativity, and empower you to make delicious and nutritious Banting-friendly meals with ease. Choose tools that align with your cooking style and preferences to enhance your Banting diet experience.

Conversion Charts and Substitution Tips

Make cooking and meal planning easier with conversion charts and substitution tips that help you adapt recipes to fit your Banting diet. These resources can assist you in making informed choices and adjustments while preparing delicious and nutritious meals:

1. Measurement Conversion Chart:

   - Use a measurement conversion chart to easily convert between different units of measurement, such as cups, ounces, grams, and milliliters. This tool is helpful for accurately measuring ingredients and following recipes from various sources.

2. Ingredient Substitution Guide:

- Refer to an ingredient substitution guide to find suitable alternatives for common ingredients that may not align with the Banting diet. For example, swap traditional flour with almond flour or coconut flour, and replace sugar with Banting-friendly sweeteners like erythritol or stevia.

3. Banting Ingredient Swaps:

- Familiarize yourself with Banting ingredient swaps to modify recipes without sacrificing flavor or texture. Substitute high-carb ingredients like potatoes, rice, or pasta with lower-carb alternatives such as cauliflower rice, zucchini noodles, or spaghetti squash.

4. Flavor Enhancers:

- Experiment with flavor enhancers and seasonings to add depth and complexity to your Banting meals. Incorporate herbs, spices, citrus zest, and aromatic vegetables like garlic and onions to elevate the taste of your dishes without relying on added sugars or unhealthy fats.

5. Healthy Fat Substitutes:

- Opt for healthy fat substitutes to replace less nutritious fats in recipes. Use avocado, olive oil, coconut oil, or ghee as alternatives to vegetable oils or butter, providing essential fatty acids and rich flavor profiles to your dishes.

6. Low-Carb Binders:

- Discover low-carb binders to thicken sauces, soups, and baked goods without using traditional starches or flours. Consider ingredients like xanthan gum, guar gum, psyllium husk powder, or gelatin as effective binding agents in Banting-friendly recipes.

7. Sweetener Conversion Chart:

- Consult a sweetener conversion chart to accurately substitute Banting-friendly sweeteners for sugar in recipes. Different sweeteners have varying levels of sweetness and may require adjustments in quantity to achieve the desired taste.

8. Allergy-Friendly Options:

- Adapt recipes to accommodate dietary restrictions or allergies by exploring allergy-friendly options and substitutions. For example, replace dairy milk with almond milk, coconut milk, or hemp milk for lactose-free alternatives in recipes.

9. Banting Baking Tips:

- Follow Banting baking tips to achieve optimal results when baking low-carb and grain-free treats. Adjust oven temperatures, baking times, and ingredient ratios to ensure successful outcomes while maintaining the integrity of Banting principles.

10. Experimentation and Adaptation:

- Embrace experimentation and adaptation in the kitchen as you explore new recipes and techniques within the Banting framework. Allow yourself to be creative and flexible, adapting recipes to suit your taste preferences and nutritional needs.

By utilizing conversion charts and substitution tips, you can confidently navigate the world of Banting cooking, make informed choices, and create delicious and satisfying meals that align with your dietary goals and preferences.

Conclusion: Embracing a Healthier Lifestyle with Banting

Transitioning to the Banting lifestyle offers numerous benefits beyond weight loss, providing a holistic approach to health and wellness. Here's how you can embrace a healthier lifestyle with Banting:

1. Focus on Whole Foods: Banting encourages the consumption of whole, unprocessed foods, such as lean proteins, healthy fats, non-starchy vegetables, and limited amounts of fruits and nuts. By prioritizing these nutrient-dense foods, you provide your body with essential vitamins, minerals, and antioxidants to support overall health and well-being.

2. Balance Macronutrients: The Banting diet emphasizes a balanced intake of macronutrients, including protein, fats, and carbohydrates. By moderating your carbohydrate intake and prioritizing healthy fats and proteins, you can stabilize blood sugar levels, improve satiety, and promote sustainable energy throughout the day.

3. Listen to Your Body: Pay attention to your body's hunger and satiety cues, and eat mindfully to foster a healthy relationship with food. Banting encourages intuitive eating, allowing you to tune into your body's signals and make food choices that nourish and satisfy you.

4. Prioritize Real Foods: Minimize the consumption of processed and refined foods that are high in sugars, additives, and unhealthy fats. Instead, opt for whole, natural foods that are minimally processed and free from artificial ingredients, supporting your body's natural functions and metabolic processes.

5. Enjoy Cooking and Meal Preparation: Embrace cooking as a creative and enjoyable activity, and take pleasure in preparing homemade meals using fresh, wholesome ingredients. Experiment with new recipes, flavors, and cooking techniques to keep your meals interesting and satisfying.

6. Stay Active: Complement your Banting lifestyle with regular physical activity to promote cardiovascular health, muscle strength, and flexibility. Engage in activities you enjoy, whether it's walking, cycling, yoga, or strength training, and strive to incorporate movement into your daily routine.

7. Practice Stress Management: Prioritize stress management techniques such as meditation, deep breathing exercises, and mindfulness to reduce stress levels and promote overall well-being. Chronic stress can negatively impact health and weight management, so finding effective coping strategies is essential.

8. Get Adequate Sleep: Prioritize quality sleep to support overall health and metabolic function. Aim for 7-9 hours of restorative sleep each night, and establish a relaxing bedtime routine to promote relaxation and prepare your body for sleep.

9. Stay Hydrated: Drink plenty of water throughout the day to stay hydrated and support optimal bodily functions. Water is essential for digestion, nutrient absorption, and the elimination of toxins, making it crucial for overall health and well-being.

10. Seek Support and Accountability: Surround yourself with a supportive community of friends, family, or fellow Banting enthusiasts who can offer encouragement, motivation, and accountability on your journey to a healthier lifestyle.

By embracing the principles of Banting and adopting a holistic approach to health and wellness, you can transform your lifestyle, improve your overall well-being, and cultivate habits that promote long-term health and vitality. Remember that progress takes time, so be patient with yourself and celebrate each step forward on your journey to a healthier you.

Celebrating Your Banting Journey

Embarking on the Banting journey is not just about changing your diet—it's about transforming your entire lifestyle and embracing a healthier way of living. As you progress on your Banting journey, it's important to celebrate your achievements and milestones along the way. Here's how you can celebrate your Banting journey:

1. Acknowledge Your Progress: Take a moment to acknowledge how far you've come since starting your Banting journey. Whether you've lost weight, improved your energy levels, or developed healthier eating habits, celebrate the progress you've made and recognize the positive changes in your life.

2. Reflect on Your Successes: Reflect on the successes and accomplishments you've achieved while following the Banting lifestyle. Celebrate the small victories, such as trying new Banting recipes, resisting temptation, or making healthier choices when dining out.

3. Share Your Achievements: Share your Banting successes with friends, family, or your Banting community. Celebrate your achievements openly and proudly, and inspire others to embark on their own journey to better health and wellness.

4. Treat Yourself: Treat yourself to something special as a reward for your hard work and dedication to the Banting lifestyle. Whether it's a new outfit, a spa day, or a fun activity you enjoy, indulge in a well-deserved reward that celebrates your commitment to health and well-being.

5. Document Your Journey: Keep a journal or diary to document your Banting journey, including your goals, challenges, and successes. Reflecting on your experiences can help you appreciate how far you've come and inspire you to continue making positive changes in your life.

6. Celebrate Non-Scale Victories: Celebrate non-scale victories that go beyond weight loss, such as improved energy levels, better sleep, clearer skin, or reduced cravings. These achievements are just as important as changes on the scale and deserve to be recognized and celebrated.

7. Host a Banting Feast: Host a Banting-friendly feast or dinner party to celebrate your progress and share your love of healthy eating with others. Prepare a delicious spread of Banting recipes and enjoy good food, laughter, and camaraderie with friends and loved ones.

8. Set New Goals: Set new goals and challenges to keep yourself motivated and inspired on your Banting journey. Whether it's trying new Banting recipes, increasing your physical activity, or mastering mindfulness techniques, set goals that align with your vision for a healthier lifestyle.

9. Practice Gratitude: Take time to practice gratitude and appreciate the abundance of health and vitality that the Banting lifestyle has brought into your life. Cultivate a mindset of gratitude for the nourishing foods, supportive community, and opportunities for growth and self-improvement that Banting has provided.

10. Celebrate Every Day: Celebrate your Banting journey every day by embracing the joy of living a healthier, happier life. Find moments of gratitude, savor delicious Banting meals, and take pride in the positive choices you make each day to prioritize your health and well-being.

By celebrating your Banting journey and embracing the positive changes it brings into your life, you can cultivate a sense of pride, fulfillment, and joy in your journey to a healthier lifestyle. Remember to celebrate every victory, big or small, and continue to nourish your body, mind, and spirit with the goodness of the Banting lifestyle.

Long-Term Success Strategies

Achieving long-term success with the Banting lifestyle involves adopting sustainable habits and strategies that support your health and well-being for the long haul. Here are some key strategies to help you maintain your progress and thrive on your Banting journey:

1. Focus on Consistency Over Perfection: Aim for consistency in your Banting habits rather than striving for perfection. While it's natural to have occasional slip-ups or indulgences, consistency in following the Banting principles over time is key to long-term success.

2. Build Healthy Habits: Establish healthy habits that support your Banting lifestyle, such as meal planning, mindful eating, regular physical activity, adequate sleep, and stress management. Consistently practicing these habits will help you maintain your progress and sustain your results over time.

3. Stay Educated and Informed: Stay informed about the latest developments and research related to the Banting lifestyle. Keep learning about nutrition, health, and wellness to deepen your understanding of how the Banting principles impact your body and overall well-being.

4. Listen to Your Body: Tune into your body's signals and listen to its cues regarding hunger, fullness, and cravings. Practice intuitive eating by eating when you're hungry, stopping when you're satisfied, and making food choices that nourish and energize you.

5. Adapt and Adjust: Be flexible and willing to adapt your Banting approach as needed based on your individual preferences, goals, and lifestyle. Experiment with different foods, recipes, and meal plans to find what works best for you, and don't be afraid to make adjustments along the way.

6. Set Realistic Goals: Set realistic and achievable goals for your Banting journey, taking into account your personal preferences, lifestyle, and circumstances. Break larger goals into smaller, manageable steps, and celebrate each milestone along the way.

7. Practice Self-Compassion: Be kind to yourself and practice self-compassion as you navigate your Banting journey. Understand that setbacks and challenges are a normal part of the process, and treat yourself with the same kindness and understanding you would offer to a friend.

8. Build a Support System: Surround yourself with a supportive network of friends, family, or fellow Banting enthusiasts who understand and encourage your goals. Lean on your support system for motivation, accountability, and encouragement during both the highs and lows of your journey.

9. Stay Engaged and Inspired: Stay engaged and inspired by connecting with the Banting community, attending events, joining online forums or social media groups, and sharing your experiences with others. Draw inspiration from success stories, recipes, and tips shared by fellow Banting enthusiasts.

10. Celebrate Your Progress: Celebrate your progress and achievements along the way, no matter how small. Take time to acknowledge your successes, express gratitude for the positive changes in your life, and reflect on how far you've come on your Banting journey.

By implementing these long-term success strategies, you can cultivate a sustainable and fulfilling Banting lifestyle that supports your health, well-being, and vitality for years to come. Embrace the journey, stay committed to your goals, and trust in your ability to thrive on the Banting path.

Final Words of Encouragement

As you embark on your journey to embrace a healthier lifestyle with Banting, remember that you are taking a significant step towards improving your overall well-being and vitality. Here are some final words of encouragement to inspire you along the way:

1. You Are Making a Positive Change: By choosing to follow the Banting lifestyle, you are making a positive change in your life that has the potential to transform your health, energy levels, and quality of life. Celebrate this decision and embrace the opportunity for growth and transformation.

2. Trust in Your Journey: Trust in the process and believe in your ability to succeed on your Banting journey. Remember that change takes time, and progress may not always be linear. Trust in your efforts, stay committed to your goals, and have faith that you are moving in the right direction.

3. Celebrate Every Victory: Celebrate every victory, no matter how small, as you progress on your Banting journey. Whether it's trying a new Banting recipe, resisting temptation, or reaching a milestone on your health and wellness goals, take time to acknowledge and celebrate your achievements along the way.

4. Stay Resilient in the Face of Challenges:
Expect challenges and setbacks to arise along your Banting journey, but don't let them deter you from your goals. Stay resilient in the face of adversity, learn from your experiences, and use them as opportunities for growth and self-improvement.

5. Find Joy in the Journey: Embrace the journey to a healthier lifestyle with Banting and find joy in the process. Enjoy experimenting with new recipes, savoring delicious and nutritious foods, and discovering the many benefits that come with prioritizing your health and well-being.

6. Stay Connected and Supported: Surround yourself with a supportive network of friends, family, or fellow Banting enthusiasts who understand and encourage your goals. Lean on your support system for motivation, accountability, and encouragement during both the highs and lows of your journey.

7. Practice Gratitude: Cultivate a mindset of gratitude for the abundance of health, vitality, and well-being that the Banting lifestyle brings into your life. Take time to appreciate the nourishing foods, supportive community, and opportunities for growth and self-discovery that you encounter along the way.

8. Remember Your Why: Reflect on your reasons for embarking on the Banting journey and stay connected to your "why" whenever you face challenges or moments of doubt. Whether it's to improve your health, boost your energy levels, or enhance your overall quality of life, keep your reasons for pursuing a healthier lifestyle at the forefront of your mind.

9. Believe in Yourself: Believe in yourself and your ability to achieve your health and wellness goals with Banting. You have the strength, determination, and resilience to overcome obstacles and create the vibrant and fulfilling life you desire.

10. You Are Worth It: Above all, remember that you are worth the effort and investment required to embrace a healthier lifestyle with Banting. Prioritize your health, well-being, and happiness, and know that you deserve to live your best life.

Embrace the journey with an open heart and a positive mindset, and trust that each step you take brings you closer to the vibrant and fulfilling life you deserve. You have the power to create lasting change and thrive on your Banting journey— believe in yourself and let your light shine brightly!